How to Lose Weight Permanently:

A Genius-Based Keys to Long-Term Weight Loss

By

Jane Rios

Table of Contents

Introduction

A positive outlook is crucial for weight loss and weight management success. You need to commit to progressively changing to a healthy lifestyle if you want to reduce weight permanently.

You must consume fewer calories daily or burn more calories than you consume to lose weight. Both are the most effective ways to lose weight.

A very low-calorie diet can make you feel deprived and increase your propensity to overeat. Very low-calorie diets frequently result in muscle loss rather than fat loss.

The result is a figure that jiggles rather than one that is toned and smooth. Exercise aids in fat loss and muscle preservation.

Extremely low-calorie diets are deficient in many essential nutrients, which increases your risk of developing malnutrition. Most importantly, data demonstrates that those who adhere to these diets typically put all the weight they lost back on. People who gradually lose weight by eating less and exercising more are more likely to keep it off.

Chapter one

Reasons for your body's excessive desire and hunger.

After eating, some people discover they are not satisfied. Dieting and thyroid issues are only two examples of the many variables that can play a role. However, occasionally, a person could experience constant hunger. Making dietary or lifestyle modifications may help a person feel less hungry. However, persistent hunger can also be a symptom of some illnesses that may require medical attention.

These are a few potential causes of constant hunger.

Dieting.

Dieting is difficult for many people because of hunger.

People on calorie-restricted diets may experience hunger all the time. Ghrelin is a hormone that the body produces when there are fewer calories consumed than are burned by the body. Because the stomach releases ghrelin when the body needs more food, some people refer to it as the "hunger hormone."

Even after a person has eaten, a low-calorie diet might stimulate ghrelin production and make them feel hungry.

Sugar-rich diet

Many foods and beverages include added sugar, which can make people feel more hungry. These imply that ingesting an excessive amount of sugar, especially fructose may cause an increase in hunger. A high-fructose diet may increase ghrelin production and alter activity in particular brain regions, which will decrease satiety. Additionally, researchers discovered that giving study participants a fructose supplement enhanced how quickly their stomachs emptied.

A diet low in protein

A person may feel less hungry if they consume more protein, according to some research.

For instance, they examined the impact of a high-protein diet on 156 obese teenagers. For three months, the individuals were randomly assigned to consume either a high-protein or low-protein breakfast. There were the same number of calories in both breakfasts.

A high-protein breakfast caused individuals to eat less at lunch and had more weight reduction and feelings of fullness than those who ate a low-protein breakfast. Adult males should ingest 56 grams (g) of protein daily, while adult females should take in 46 g.

Instead of consuming it all at once, it may help to consume some protein with each meal or snack.

Dehydration

It's crucial to drink enough water to stay healthy. A person may feel more satisfied if they drink water, according to some data. For instance, the impact of excessive water consumption in overweight women. The women reported having less appetite and losing weight after 8 weeks.

Fiber-poor diet

Dietary fiber is crucial for a healthy digestive system, reducing constipation, and may also help you feel fuller for longer.

In comparison to those who took a placebo, individuals who took psyllium fiber supplements felt less hungry in between meals. The same was true for those who consumed a maltodextrin fiber supplement. It is advised that:

Males aged 19 to 50 consume 38 g of fiber each day.

Women between the ages of 19 and 50 consume 25 g of fiber daily.

Sleep disturbance.

Getting adequate sleep can support hormone levels that are in a healthy range.

The body's natural hormonal balance can be upset by not getting enough sleep, which may make some people feel more hungry.
Obesity and diabetes are only two of the health concerns that research has connected sleep disruption to. Men who slept less than usual had greater ghrelin levels and consumed more calories.

Boredom

Some people could mistake hunger for boredom and overeat as a result. When someone is bored, they may turn to rewarding activities like eating.

Salt-heavy diet

The typical American consumes more than 3,400 mg of sodium per day, the majority of which comes from processed foods. The recommended daily sodium intake is 2,300 mg, however, most adults should strive to consume less than 1,500 mg. But salty meals might have an impact on more than just heart health.

Consuming a lot of salt can make a person eat more. For instance, involving 48 healthy adults discovered that those who ate high-salt meals consumed more calories than those who ate low-salt meals.

Menopause

Females going through menopause have a higher risk of gaining weight. Numerous causes, including hormone changes, may be to blame for this medication
The loss of estrogen hormones during menopause may cause an increase in hunger.

Medications

The metabolism and hunger signals of the body can be impacted by some drugs. Some antidepressants, antipsychotics, and corticosteroids can make someone feel more ravenous than usual. Anyone who has taken a new drug and gained a lot of weight should talk to their doctor. They may suggest lowering the dosage or switching to a different medication, or they may offer advice on coping mechanisms.

Resistance to leptin

A hormone called leptin alerts the brain when the stomach is full. After a meal, leptin levels normally increase. When the body does not react to leptin as it should, this condition is known as leptin resistance. As a result, after eating a meal, a person might not feel satisfied. Leptin resistance is a common condition in overweight or obese people, which can lead to increased hunger.

Stress

Emotional stress and issues with eating control are related, according to research on stress. These discovered that those under stress from marital problems had higher ghrelin levels and a lower-quality diet than individuals in more stable relationships.

Synthetic sweeteners

Artificial sweeteners are added by manufacturers to a variety of goods, including diet sodas and foods with no or little added sugar. These sugar replacements can assist a person in consuming less sugar overall.

Artificial sweeteners, however, may stimulate the appetite, according to research conducted on animals For instance, a diet sweetened with the common artificial sweetener sucralose

Drinking alcohol

Alcohol use could make you hungry. Alcohol use has the potential to increase hunger.

These indicate that the association between drinking and overeating may result from alcohol's impact on the brain's hunger signals. Participants who drank alcohol before a meal were more aware of the scents of the food and consumed more.

Breastfeeding

Breastfeeding mothers need more calories to create milk, which could boost their appetite. 450–500 more calories are consumed each day by nursing mothers.

Unbalanced thyroid

A little gland called the thyroid can be seen near the front of the neck. It creates hormones that regulate metabolism and the body's energy usage. There are many signs of hyperthyroidism, or an overactive thyroid, including increased hunger.

A bloated neck, weight loss, feeling hot, diarrhea, irritability, anxiousness, mood swings, weariness, hyperactivity, and more frequent urination are some other signs of hyperthyroidism. With a physical examination and a blood test, a doctor can typically identify hyperthyroidism. Medication, radioiodine therapy, and thyroid surgery are available as treatments.

Diabetes type 2

Type 2 diabetes might cause persistent hunger. Diabetes prevents glucose from entering cells, which use glucose as a source of energy, and instead keeps it in the blood.

A person could become hungry and exhausted as a result.

Increased thirst, frequent urination, eyesight issues, slower wound and cut healing, and unexplained weight loss are other signs of type 2 diabetes. People who exhibit type 2 diabetes symptoms should visit a doctor for a diagnosis. A quick blood test can frequently identify diabetes in a patient. Medication, nutritional, and lifestyle modifications are all possible forms of treatment.

A person may experience constant hunger for a variety of reasons. By changing their diets to include more protein and fiber, eating less sugar and salt, drinking more water, restricting processed or fried foods, and drinking less alcohol, they may be able to lessen this appetite. Some drugs may have a side effect that makes you feel more hungry. However, it may also be a sign of a medical problem, such as type 2 diabetes, stress, or hyperthyroidism. People who have unexplained weight loss or persistent hunger should think about consulting a doctor.

Chapter two

Emotional Eating:

Emotional eating is the tendency of one sufferer to respond to stressful, difficult feelings by eating, even when not experiencing physical hunger. Emotional eating or emotional hunger is craving for high-calorie or high-carbohydrate foods that have small nutritional value often. The foods that emotional eaters crave are often referred to as comfort foods, such as ice cream, cookies, chocolate, chips, French fries, and pizza. Consequently, stress can be related with both weight gain and weight loss. Binge eating disorder is a distinctive mental illness that causes a series of compulsive overeating, the affected people uncontrollably eat an amount of food that is larger than that which most people eat in a distinct period for over two hours, even when they are not hungry. It's seen in girls and women being at higher risk for eating disorders, showing they are at higher risk for emotional eating. However, men are more likely to eat in response to depression or anger, and women are more likely to eat excessively in response to failing a diet. Some people whose their emotions cause them to eat may have been raised to connect food with feelings instead of sustenance, particularly if the food was often used as a reward or punishment, or as a substitute for emotional intimacy.

Emotional eaters like unhealthy foods, due to an unpleasant emotion of some type, such as stress, boredom, sadness, anger, guilt, or frustration.

Other characteristics of emotional eating include a loss of control during eating.

Emotional eating is diagnosed.

The patient must first undergo a physical examination and lab tests to rule out the possibility that the symptom is a result of a genetic or other medical illness, such as Prader-Willi syndrome before they are diagnosed To distinguish between emotional eating and other eating disorders like bulimia, binge eating, or pica, a detailed investigation of any history of mental health symptoms will be made. If further types of mental disease are present, a mental health professional will look at it as well.

Treatments for emotional eating.

Understanding one's triggers for indulging in this behavior, learning healthier ways to perceive food, adopting better eating habits, and creating effective stress management strategies are all common steps in overcoming emotional eating.

Exercise is a crucial component of stress management since it has been shown to reduce the release of stress hormones, which can reduce symptoms of anxiety, sleeplessness, and depression as well as the propensity for emotional eating.

Another way for managing stress and reducing emotional eating is to practice meditation and other relaxation techniques.

Other crucial strategies for effectively managing stress include abstaining from drugs and alcohol and only ingesting modest amounts of each. This is because many of these substances intensify the body's reaction to stress. Additionally, abusing those substances frequently stops the person from confronting their issues head-on, making it difficult for them to come up with efficient stress-reduction or stress-eradication strategies.

Taking breaks at home and the office are other lifestyle modifications that help reduce stress. Avoid scheduling yourself too much. Recognize your stress triggers and learn how to handle them.

Take regular days off at the appropriate times. Create a comfortable response to the unexpected by organizing your life. Stress-management counseling in the form of individual or group therapy can be quite beneficial for persons who may require assistance managing their stress. It has been demonstrated that stress counseling and group therapy can lessen the symptoms of stress and enhance general health.

Assisting the person in altering the way they view specific circumstances, this method helps to reduce stress. To achieve these objectives employs this techniques:

Cognitive component: This aids in identifying the beliefs and presumptions that affect a person's actions, particularly those that might make a person more likely to engage in emotional eating. Teaching mindfulness and being present in the moment without judgment is a variant of the cognitive therapy approach. Mindfulness entails thinking more critically, raising emotional intelligence, and improving one's capacity to distinguish between feelings and hunger.

behavioral element The person is taught how to quit emotional eating and apply better problem-solving approaches through the use of behavior-modification techniques.

Selective serotonin reuptake inhibitors (SSRIs), in particular, can be very helpful if stress results in severe mental issues like post-traumatic stress disorder (PTSD), clinical depression, or anxiety disorders. Sertraline (Zoloft), paroxetine (Paxil), fluoxetine (Prozac), citalopram (Celexa), and escitalopram (Lexapro) are a few SSRI examples.

However, compared to persons who prefer to eat less while under stress, those who are prone to emotional eating are also frequently more responsive to stress reduction in reversing their predisposition to do so.

Emotional eating prevention.

Reducing stress, utilizing healthy methods of understanding and managing emotions, and viewing food as nourishment rather than a means of solving problems

Practicing meditation, working out, and other healthy stress reduction and stress management practices, abstaining from much coffee, alcohol, and narcotics, are additional ways to prevent emotional eating behaviors.

Chapter three.

Reasons you Love Eating Unhealthy Foods.

Despite its ugly name, many people love junk food. Why? it's super available, inexpensive, and made to hit your taste buds in a way that makes you crave more and more of it.

WHAT IS JUNK FOOD?

"Junk" food is the unhealthy food we eat that has little nutritional value making it high in empty calories like Candy, chips, cookies, cake, sugary soft drinks, French fries, ice cream, and most things served at fast food places. While there's a place for everything in a healthy diet, eating too much of this kind of food can cause weight gain and other health risks. Knowing more about what makes unhealthy food so tempting may help you to limit how much you eat it.

Junk food is so Appealing

There are reasons why less healthy foods especially those so-called "junk" foods are so popular, even though we know they are not the best choice for health and well-being.

It's Affordable

Most junk food is cheap. You can go to any fast food place and order something off a dollar menu of some sort. It's no different at the food store. Inexpensive snacks and high-sodium, high-fat meals with low price tags are easily available. Healthier foods like fresh fruits and veggies have a reputation for being costlier, though they say this is not always the case.

Keep in mind that fresh conventional and even organic produce is beginning to become more affordable. Although a lot of junk food may seem cheap to buy upfront, the case can be made that junk foods end up being more expensive in the long run due to their negative impact on health.

It's Easily Seen.

Junky snack foods lurk in vending machines, convenience stores, and the check-out lanes of supermarkets, big-box retailers, and even office-supply stores and other places that don't usually sell food items. And those instant meals earlier mentioned? They're easy to prepare, and you can stockpile them in your cooking cabinet for a long time.

Of course, fast foods live up to the name, You can order a fast-food meal and then eat it a minute or two later. You don't even have to get out of your car.

It's Tasty, Salty and Fatty.

Rarely do junk foods tempt you with delicate or difficult flavors. They will hit you hard with sweetness, fat, and salt. Picky eaters may prefer these simpler flavors—it could be slightly bitter taste of many vegetables turns some people off, especially kids.

But it's more than taste. Various mixtures of sugar and fat make for textures people like. Fat makes things smooth and creamy, like ice cream and butter. Starchy potato and corn chips cooked in hot oil have a pleasant salty crunch.

That's to say that nutrient-dense foods aren't appealing, but sometimes the textures of fresh fruits and veggies is hard getting used to if you tend to consume a lot of processed foods.

It's a habit

Because junk foods are easy to find, easy to make, and a lot of them just flat-out taste good, eating them becomes a habit.

Eating a sweet bar now and then or enjoying a bag of fries on occasion can all be part of a well-rounded diet. But when you crave junk foods, and they make up a big part of your daily diet, you run the risk of becoming overweight and fat. Plus, you're not going to get enough of the nutrients and carbohydrates your body needs for good health.

The next time you find yourself standing in line at a burger joint, think about how your choice could affect your health, and consider making some changes.

Chapter Four

Creating Your Diet Plan for Weight Loss

A well-planned eating strategy is necessary to lose weight in a significant and permanent way. For sustained energy throughout workouts and daily activities, the body requires a proper ratio of calories and nutrition. The reason of losing fat and keeping it off over time is to retain that equilibrium.

The vitamins and minerals the body requires to retain energy and develop muscle are included in a practical and delicious cuisine in an effective weight-loss diet plan. To create a diet plan for weight loss that is specially tailored to match your lifestyle, objectives, and habits, follow these steps.

Avoid much intake of calories Diet Programmes

Common diet regimens specify a daily calorie target. Dieters are required to stick to a daily intake range and eat meals that are full of the essential nutrients their bodies require to flourish. But many dieters are already doomed to failure by this fundamental tenet. We advise a whole different strategy for calorie counting. Why is counting calories every day the wrong way to think about dietary intake?

Each food has a unique number of calories. It becomes challenging to monitor your intake without tedious tracking unless you eat nearly the same thing every day.

There are certain occasions when dieters simply can't maintain a tight daily count without giving up the enjoyment of social circumstances, like going out with friends or traveling on vacation.

Many diet regimens call for a "cheat day" where the dieter is allowed to eat anything they want without monitoring calories to avoid temptation. Due to one weekly day of indulgence, it is possible to follow a daily restrictive calorie count and still fail to lose weight.

Dieters strive to maintain calorie deficits by staying within their limitations. Too many calories missing have a detrimental cumulative effect on weight loss efforts.

We advise you to create a diet plan that addresses your nutritional needs to maintain a healthy lifestyle rather than putting yourself in a daily calorie limit. This strategy is quite beneficial for weight loss since it boosts your energy levels, is less strenuous, and allows you to indulge in whatever you want as long as you do so in moderation. Everybody has their various dietary requirements depending on their age, weight, degree of activity, and other medical requirements. Eat a range of meals to achieve weight loss objectives by setting these nutritional goals or standards. These dietary objectives are centered on your intake of protein, carbohydrates, fats, vitamins, and minerals. A more effective strategy for weight loss than counting calories is maintaining these important components in balance with what your body requires.

Examine your macros.

Make sure you are providing your body with the nutrients it requires to maintain a high level of energy, burn fat, and build muscle. The fundamental building elements that your body requires to carry out these jobs are known as macronutrients. The majority of your daily calories come from these basic nutrients. The following are the three main types of macros:

Carbohydrates. To fuel muscles, simple and complex sugar chains are broken down in the body.

Fats. To supply emergency energy when quick-burning carbohydrates are not accessible, extra calories are stored in fat cells. Additionally, many hormones and brain processes depend on fat.

Proteins. The body's tissues can heal and grow as a result of the material and energy that these powerful macros supply.

You have the best chance of developing the body you want without feeling starved or worn out if you balance these macronutrients.

The typical recommendation is that you should consume 35% healthy fat, 40% protein, and 25% carbohydrates each day. Use an online calculator to find your ideal combination for a more customized ratio.

Know the Foods that fit in

Find meals that work with your new lifestyle after you've determined how much to consume. You must include things that you'll consume in your diet plan if you want to lose weight. It's doubtful that you will follow your plan if you don't appreciate the food you're eating.

But it's also crucial to make an effort to explore different menu choices.

Due to a restrictive diet high in empty calories, many dieters enroll in weight loss programs. In developing a long-term eating strategy one needs to increase the number of nutritious selections on your daily menu.

Make a list of your favorite dishes and ingredients to get started.

Once you start eating healthy, try adding one or two new fruits, vegetables, or grains to your list each week. It's useful to check information on each item's macronutrient content because you can use the information to determine how much of each ingredient you can eat at each meal.

Save up your recipes.

Now that you are aware of what you can eat, begin gathering a range of recipes that use the ingredients you have identified. The amount of macronutrients in your food is greatly influenced by how you prepare it.

Your diet plan for weight loss should include a variety of recipes that interest you and prevent boredom. The main reason many dieters fail to accomplish their objectives is that they grow bored with their everyday diets.

You can modify your recipe collection to suit your preferences if you do enough study. Are sweetbreads and pastries your favorite foods? Your favorite baked items may be found in low-calorie varieties. Are sauces a crucial component of your regular meals? Look for handmade versions of the condiments you use the most. Do you feel anxious about giving up fried foods? Look for recipes that can imitate the crisp you crave in the oven without adding extra oil.

Make a list of the restaurants you go to the most often if you're someone who is constantly on the go. Inquire about the menu items' nutritional information from the staff. Utilize the information to compile a list of options that are under your dietary spending limit.

Plan your Mealtime

Just as crucial as what you eat is when you eat.

Our capacity to metabolize stomach contents is impacted by daily cycles that occur in our bodies. In addition, pre-existing medical issues or variations in how your body functions can affect how you metabolize food.

A diet plan for weight loss that adheres to the conventional paradigm of three meals per day often fails. This is particularly valid for those actively reducing their daily caloric consumption. Try to separate your meals and snacks by around three hours. This prevents you from becoming overly hungry and turning to bad foods to satisfy your needs. Here are some additional suggestions to assist you in creating the ideal food program for weight loss.

Avoid late-night snacks, eat a substantial dinner.

Eat a breakfast heavy in protein within an hour of waking up.

Keep to the meals you have planned.

Consult your doctor for assistance in creating a routine that supports maintaining the right blood sugar levels if you have diabetes or other glucose issues that are affected by your eating habits.

Refine and Examine

To keep track of your meal plan, use a food journal. This establishes a record that enables you to review your eating patterns and enable the success of your strategy.

Chapter Five.

How to Keep Off Weight Permanently

You may be familiar with the frequently cited statistic that 95% of dieters who lose weight will gain it back within a few years—or even months. This is because excessively restrictive diets are difficult to maintain over time. That doesn't mean that your efforts to lose weight will fail. Not at all.

Now that you've finally reached the magic number, what should you do? The objective is to shed the additional weight and keep it off forever. Sadly, only approximately a third of dieters are successful in keeping off their weight loss. Veteran dieters are aware that maintaining weight reduction requires vigilance, which for some people is harder than losing the weight itself.

Continued lifestyle change is necessary to maintain weight loss. Weight gain is unavoidable if you resume the behaviors that made you overweight in the first place.

Similar to the habits you formed when you were losing weight, a good diet and exercise routines are required for permanent weight loss. After losing weight, many people lose too much weight and then quickly regain it. Once you've accomplished your aim, you can begin to unwind a little, but only a little.

Over 10,000 people who dropped a considerable amount of weight and kept it off for extended periods have been followed by this. Whatever diet you initially follow, forming these routines may help you keep the weight off:

Continue to be active. Successful dieters often walk for 60 minutes of exercise.

Log your meals. Making a daily food journal will help you stay accountable and inspired.

Daily breakfast is a must. Typically, it consists of cereal and fruit. Consume less bad fat and more fiber than you would in the average American diet.

Check the scale often. You may be able to see any slight weight gains by weighing yourself once a week, which will allow you to act quickly before the issue worsens.

Watch less TV shows. Reducing the amount of time you spend in front of a screen while eating can help you live a more active lifestyle and avoid gaining weight.

Practice Leads to Perfection

Something becomes simpler the more you do it. Making such good habits a routine requires time. Don't allow all your hard work to go to waste; be patient with yourself. Recognize your areas of weakness and be ready. There will be times when you'll feel tempted by particular meals or circumstances, but if your resolve is strong, you can resist temptations. The best strategy in those challenging circumstances is moderation.

One of my favorite weight-maintenance techniques is to designate a day of the week when I can indulge a little. This day must change from week to week;

otherwise, you can end up having more than one "off" day per week as a result of the situation. I allow myself to treat myself to my favorite meals on my scheduled day off, which is usually a Saturday for obvious reasons. It's okay to have a small cheesecake slice, but not the entire thing! In essence, it is deliberate cheating. It works a treat for me, and it might be for you as well. Even just knowing that I can relax on Saturday helps me perform well all week.

It gets simpler to maintain the loss the longer people keep the weight off. Successful losers enjoy their new lifestyles, and leading a healthy existence no longer feels like a hardship. It must be a way of life rather than just a diet.

And it does grow simpler with time to maintain weight. Most likely, you're in the clear if you can make it to two years.

Maintain Your Course

Maintain your drive and don't allow obstacle derail you: Simply get back up after falling off the wagon and carry on with your winning strategy. You can maintain your weight indefinitely if you can train your brain to think and behave like a thin person. Additionally, it gets simpler the more you practice. By the time you reach the maintenance level, likely, you've already discovered patterns, methods, and abilities that have helped you stay on course.

Gratify yourself. You should be commended for making positive dietary and activity adjustments that not only inspire your loved ones but also have a major positive impact on your health.

According to research, long-term weight maintenance is correlated with staying in touch with the individuals or programs that assisted you in losing weight. Maintaining contact with those who gave you the initial boost to success makes sense. Stay put and let them assist you in keeping off the weight!